State Indicator Report
on Physical Activity, 2014

What is the report

The *State Indicator Report on Physical Activity, 2014,* presents state-level information on physical activity behaviors and on environmental and policy supports for physical activity.

What is already known

People who are physically active generally live longer and have a lower risk for heart disease, stroke, type 2 diabetes, depression, some cancers, and obesity. Environmental and policy strategies such as access to safe places for physical activity, physical education and physical activity in schools and child care settings, and street-scale and community-scale design policy can help increase physical activity behavior among all Americans.

What are the key findings

This report shows that physical activity among adults and high school students is higher in some states than others. Overall, most states have environmental and policy strategies in place that encourage physical activity.

How can this report be used

The *State Indicator Report on Physical Activity, 2014,* can be used to illustrate how states support physical activity and identify opportunities to improve access to environmental supports such as sidewalks or walking paths for active behavior.

What are the implications for public health practice

State health departments can work with governmental and non-governmental partners to create safe places for physical activity, to enhance physical education and physical activity in schools and child care settings, and to support street-scale and community-scale design policy. These partnerships will likely depend on the type of activities a state chooses to focus on. For example, some state departments of health, parks and recreation, and education may work together to help communities establish joint-use agreements that allow residents to use school physical activity facilities after school hours. To increase residents' access to safe sidewalks, state departments of health, transportation, and community organization may work together to support street-scale design policies.

Being physically active is one of the most important steps that Americans can take to improve their health. The *2008 Physical Activity Guidelines for Americans* recommends that adults participate in at least 2 hours and 30 minutes (150 minutes) a week of moderate-intensity aerobic physical activity and at least two or more times a week of muscle-strengthening activities for health benefits.[1] For additional and more extensive health benefits, adults should increase their aerobic physical activity to 300 minutes (5 hours) a week of moderate intensity.[1] Children and adolescents should do 1 hour (60 minutes) or more of physical activity daily.[1]

People who are physically active generally live longer and have a lower risk for heart disease, stroke, type 2 diabetes, depression, and some cancers.[2] Physical activity can also help control weight.[2] However, only about half of adults and less than a third of youth meet aerobic physical activity guidelines.[3,4] To improve physical activity behaviors among residents, state health departments, other state and local government agencies, and their partners can work together to implement the Community Preventive Services Task Force's recommended environmental and policy strategies for increasing physical activity. These strategies include 1) Creating or enhancing access to safe places for physical activity; 2) Enhancing physical education and physical activity in schools and child care settings; and 3) Supporting street-scale and community-scale design policy.

The *State Indicator Report on Physical Activity, 2014,* provides information for each state on state-level supports for the three environmental and policy strategies listed above for increasing physical activity and physical activity behaviors. This report, which can be used to inform decision makers throughout the state, shows that physical activity among adults and youth is higher in some states than others; and overall, most states have environmental supports such as sidewalks or walking paths in place that encourage physical activity. Additionally, the three "Stories from the Field" included in the report highlight efforts by state or local health agencies and their partners to implement initiatives that help increase physical activity behavior among residents.

This report shows that many state health departments, other state and local government agencies, and their partners are working to improve access and establish polices that make it easier to be physically active in communities and schools. For example, 27 states have created state-level Complete Streets policies that help to ensure that streets are safe for all users including pedestrians and bicyclists. In addition, 34 states provide guidance on policies for school districts or schools on walking or biking to or from school.

However, more work needs to be done to increase access to opportunities to be physically active. Only 20 states provide guidance to districts or school staff on establishing joint-use agreements. No states have child care regulations that fully align with national standards for moderate- to vigorous-intensity physical activity for preschoolers. Additionally, nearly half of youth live in neighborhoods without parks or playgrounds, community centers, and walking paths or sidewalks.

Many actors, however, play a role in improving physical activity and supports for physical activity. State health departments can continue to work with other state and local governmental and non-governmental agencies to create or enhance access to safe places for physical activity, enhance physical education and physical activity in schools and child care settings, and support street- and community-scale design policies.

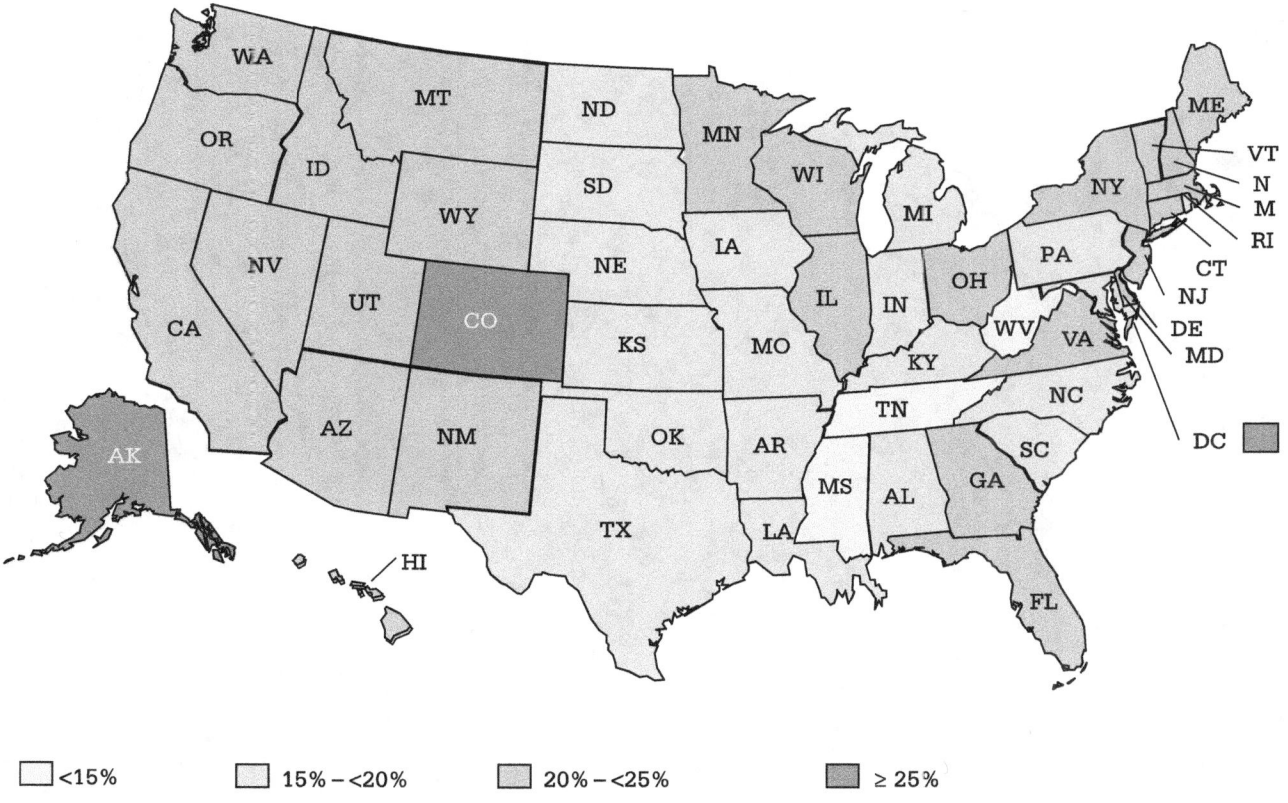

Stories from the Field

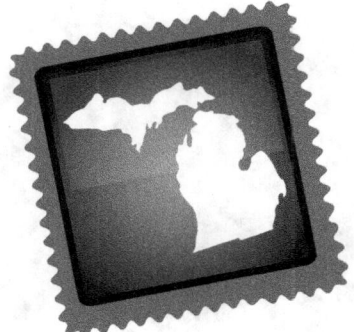

The Michigan Department of Community Health's Complete Streets Initiative included statewide efforts to educate and promote the need for local Complete Streets ordinances. Community members who witnessed the effects of local Complete Streets ordinances supported the statewide Complete Streets measure. Michigan policymakers introduced and adopted a statewide Complete Streets resolution.

After two years of work, the state-level Complete Streets legislation was passed on August 1, 2010. Under this legislation, the Michigan Department of Transportation will consider all legal users of the roads, from public transportation riders and motorists, to bicyclists and pedestrians when considering transportation design. As of 2013, at least thirty-eight Complete Streets policies have been implemented throughout the state and more than two million Michigan residents live in a community with a Complete Streets resolution or ordinance.

State-level Complete Streets policies formalize a state's intent to plan, design, and maintain streets so they are safe for all users of all ages and abilities.

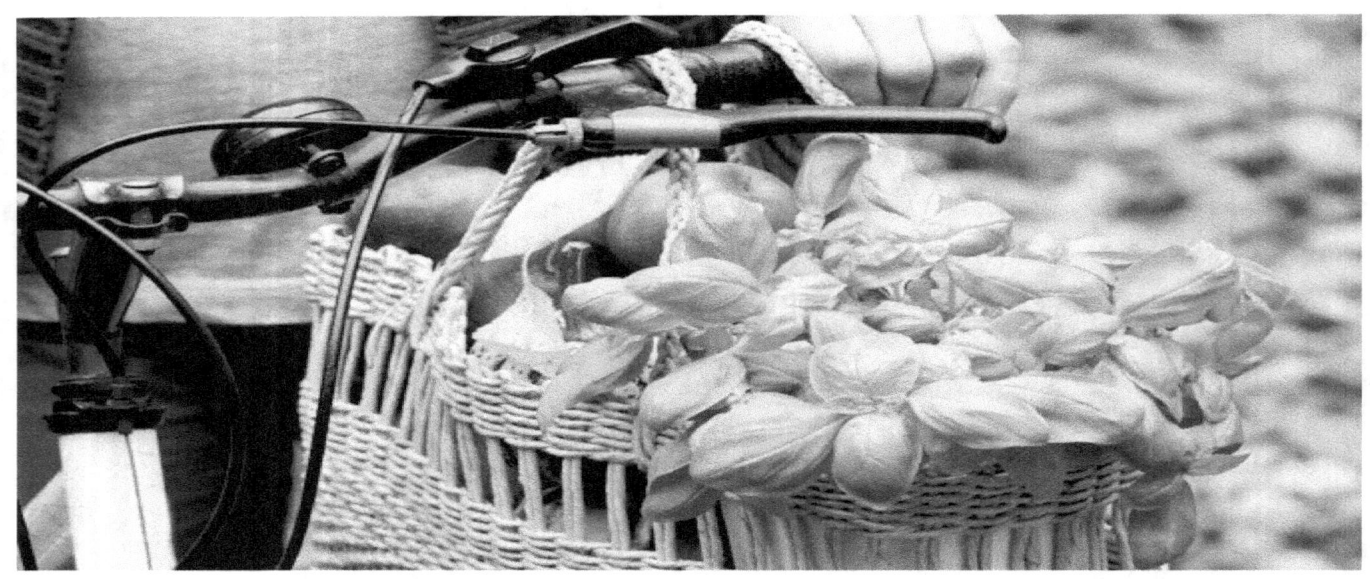

Boston
Bike-to-Market Program

The Bike-to-Market program in Boston, Massachusetts is a community health program established by bicyclist organizations, public health researchers, and city representatives. The program provides opportunities for community members to safely ride bikes for transportation. The program also encourages Boston residents to bike to famers' markets.

The Bike-to-Market program increased local access to bicycles for Bostonians, decreased bicycle theft, improved cyclists' knowledge about bicycle safety, and increased civic engagement in street redesigns for bicycle and pedestrian safety. The program bridged community interests in bicycling as transportation with access to farmers' markets by providing free bike services to children and adults at various farmers' markets in Boston neighborhoods that lack a bicycle repair shop. These included services such as bicycle repair, safety equipment and education, and bicycle lock distribution.

Since the Bike-to-Market program began in 2010, it has repaired over 1,600 bicycles and expanded the program from 9 to 16 farmers' markets. By the end of the 2011 farmers' market season, 265 helmets were distributed to program participants. In 2012, based on community input at Bike-to-Market stands, the Boston Cyclists Union, an organization that fosters collaboration among Boston cyclists groups to promote better cycling in neighborhoods, began promoting indoor bike parking at affordable housing developments to reduce bike theft and making bicycling easier in low-income communities.

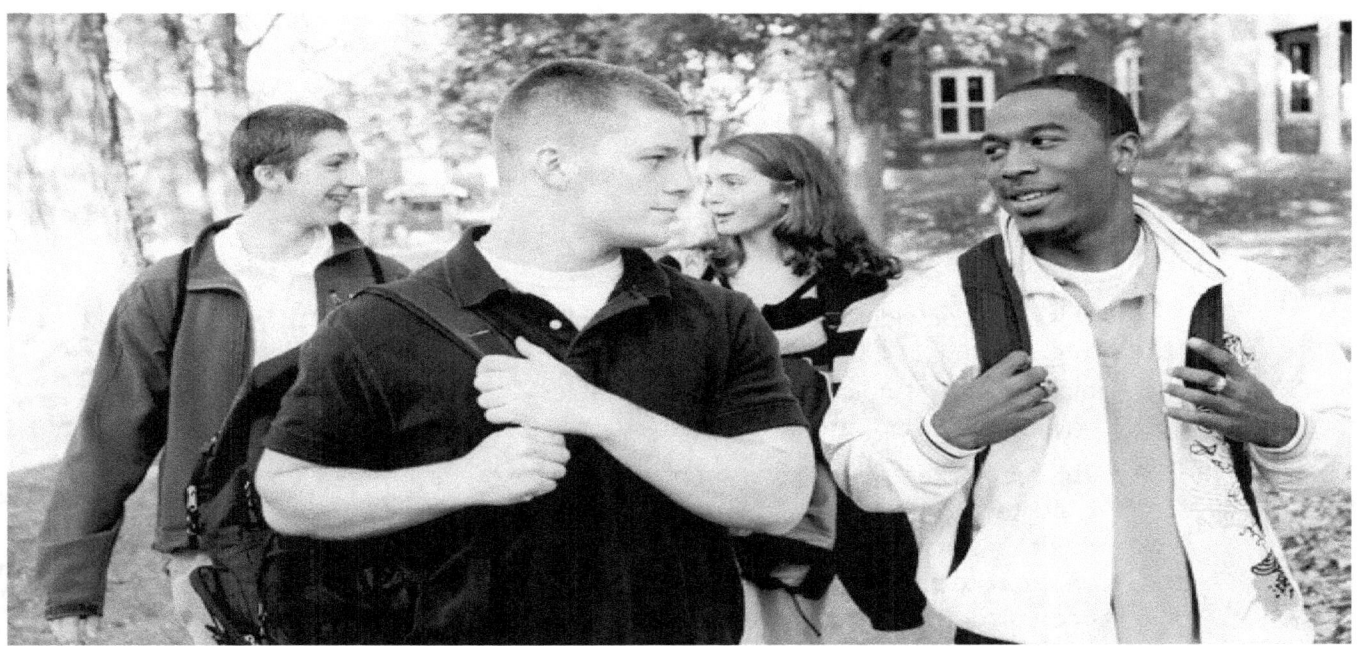

Minnesota
Safe Routes to School

The Statewide Health Improvement Program (SHIP) is a Minnesota Department of Health initiative to help Minnesota residents live longer, healthier lives by reducing the burden of chronic disease. This program supports activities such as staffing, trainings, and partnership engagement for Safe Routes to School.

The Minnesota Department of Health convened a Safe Routes to School committee within its Active Living Advisory Group to support statewide activities related to Safe Routes to School. Minnesota hired an Active Transportation Coordinator to focus solely on Safe Routes to School. The coordinator's efforts increased collaboration between the departments of Health, Education, and Transportation. With input from the Safe Routes to School committee, the Minnesota

Department of Health developed a statewide training for communities implementing active living strategies to promote regular physical activity, including Safe Routes to School.

Through Minnesota's Statewide Health Improvement Program, 181 schools that serve over 79,000 students have implemented Safe Routes to School or walking school bus policies.

Physical Activity Indicators

This report provides data on behavioral, policy, and environmental indicators for 50 states and the District of Columbia ("states"). There are nine behavioral indicators presented in Table 1 and eight policy and environmental indicators presented in Table 2.

This report presents indicators of physical activity behaviors that are consistent with the *2008 Physical Activity Guidelines for Americans,* guidelines that help Americans improve their health through appropriate physical activity, and *Healthy People 2020,* a description of our nation's health priorities. The indicators profile the extent to which adults and youth achieve these guidelines and objectives. The report uses data from Centers for Disease Control and Prevention's (CDC) Behavioral Risk Factor Surveillance System, U.S. Census Bureau's American Community Survey, and CDC's Youth Risk Behavior Surveillance System to track state-level physical activity behaviors. Tracking behavior of physical activity over time will help states monitor progress toward increased physical activity among its population. There are 9 behavioral indicators for adults and youth. The boxes on the next page reflect those indicators.

Behavioral Indicators

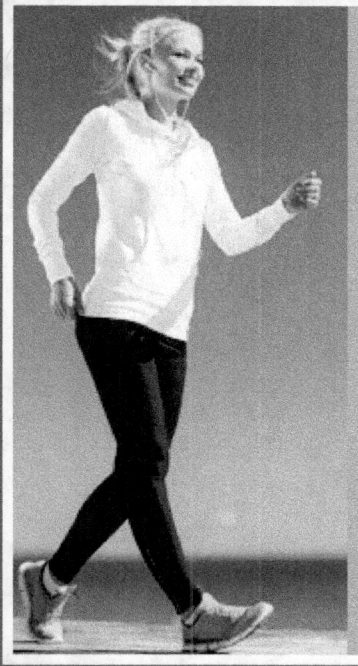

Adult Behavioral Indicators

- Percentage of adults in the state who engaged in no leisure-time physical activity
- Percentage of adults in the state who met the 150 minute aerobic activity guideline
- Percentage of adults in the state who met the 300 minute aerobic activity guideline
- Percentage of adults in the state who met the muscle-strengthening guideline
- Percentage of adults in the state who met the 150 minute aerobic activity guideline and the muscle-strengthening guideline
- Percentage of adults in the state who usually biked or walked to work in the last week

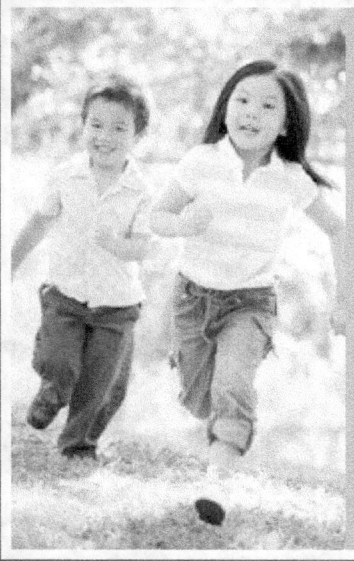

Youth Behavioral Indicators

- Percentage of students in grades 9–12 in the state who did not engage in at least 60 minutes of physical activity on any day
- Percentage of students in grades 9–12 in the state who met the aerobic activity guideline
- Percentage of students in grades 9–12 in the state who engaged in daily school physical education

2008 Physical Activity Guidelines for Americans

Key Guidelines for Adults

- All adults should avoid inactivity. Some physical activity is better than none, and adults who participate in any amount of physical activity gain some health benefits.

- For substantial health benefits, adults should do at least 150 minutes (2 hours and 30 minutes) a week of moderate intensity, or 75 minutes (1 hour and 15 minutes) a week of vigorous-intensity aerobic physical activity, or an equivalent combination of moderate- and vigorous-intensity aerobic activity. Aerobic activity should be performed in episodes of at least 10 minutes, and preferably, it should be spread throughout the week.

- For additional and more extensive health benefits, adults should increase their aerobic physical activity to 300 minutes (5 hours) a week of moderate intensity, or 150 minutes a week of vigorous intensity aerobic physical activity, or an equivalent combination of moderate- and vigorous-intensity activity. Additional health benefits are gained by engaging in physical activity beyond this amount.

- Adults should also do muscle-strengthening activities that are moderate or high intensity and involve all major muscle groups on 2 or more days a week, as these activities provide additional health benefits.

Key Guidelines for Youth and Children

- Children and adolescents should do 60 minutes (1 hour) or more of physical activity daily.

  ◊ **Aerobic:** Most of the 60 or more minutes a day should be either moderate- or vigorous-intensity aerobic physical activity, and should include vigorous-intensity physical activity at least 3 days a week.

  ◊ **Muscle-strengthening:** As part of their 60 or more minutes of daily physical activity, children and adolescents should include muscle-strengthening physical activity on at least 3 days of the week.

  ◊ **Bone-strengthening:** As part of their 60 or more minutes of daily physical activity, children and adolescents should include bone-strengthening physical activity on at least 3 days of the week.

- It is important to encourage young people to participate in physical activities that are appropriate for their age, that are enjoyable, and that offer variety.

Changes to State-Level Surveillance Systems Used to Track Physical Activity: Behavioral Risk Factor Surveillance System and Youth Risk Behavioral Surveillance System Updates

In 2011, the two surveillance systems used to track state-level physical activity behaviors, Behavioral Risk Factor Surveillance System (BRFSS) and Youth Risk Behavioral Surveillance System (YRBSS), made changes to their surveys that impacted state physical activity estimates. The physical activity estimates from the BRFSS were updated in two ways. First, there was an overall change in the BRFSS methodology to adjust sample weighting procedures and accommodate cell phone usage. Second, there were changes to the core questions to assess physical activity. Because of these changes, estimates of adult physical activity from 2011 forward cannot be compared to estimates from previous years. Data estimates from BRFSS collected in 2011 will provide a new baseline for physical activity in subsequent years. The YRBSS physical activity estimates were updated by changing the questions used to assess adolescent physical activity in 2011. Therefore, estimates of physical activity from the 2011 YRBSS provide new baseline data for youth. Youth bone- and muscle-strengthening data are not collected by YRBSS or any other state-based surveillance system and thus, not included in this report.

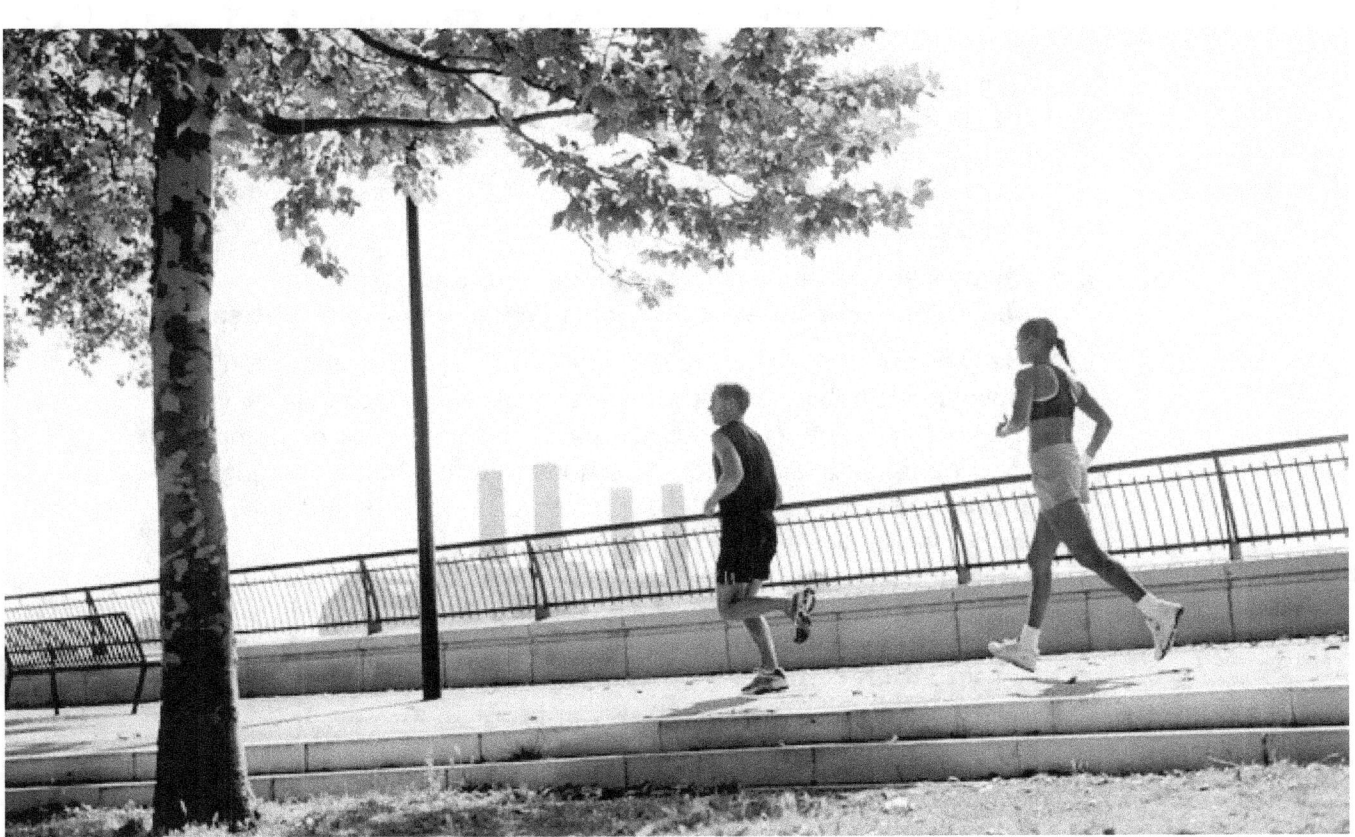

Policy and Environmental Indicators

In addition to physical activity behavior indicators, this report presents policy and environmental indicators for physical activity in each state. The 8 policy and environmental indicators* described below reflect 3 overarching strategies to increase physical activity. The 3 strategies are:

1. **Create or enhance access to safe places for physical activity;**

2. **Enhance physical education and physical activity in schools and child care settings; and**

3. **Support street-scale and community-scale design policy.**

Each strategy is supported by *The CDC Guide to Strategies for Increasing Physical Activity in the Community,*[5] *The Guide for Community Preventive Services,*[6] and *The National Physical Activity Plan.*[7] These 3 strategies can be supported at the state level as well as at the local level in communities across the state. States may choose to focus on improving some or all of the 8 indicators based on their capacity, partnerships, and resources.

1. Create or Enhance Access to Safe Places for Physical Activity

People may have the necessary knowledge, skills, attitudes, and motivation to be physically active, but if they do not have access to the necessary places where they can be active, they may be restricted or prohibited from being physically active.[5] Opportunities and environmental supports that create or enhance access to safe places for physical activity may include improving neighborhood access to quality parks, sidewalks, walking paths, or local physical activity facilities.

State provides guidance on policies for school districts or schools on joint-use agreements for physical activity facilities

A *Healthy People 2020* objective (PA-10) is to increase the proportion of the nation's public and private schools that provide access to their physical activity spaces and facilities for all persons outside of normal school hours (e.g., before and after school, on weekends, and during summer and other vacations).[8] This access to indoor and outdoor facilities for physical activity supports increased physical activity participation among community members.[9]

Percentage of youth in a state with parks or playground areas; recreation centers, community centers or boys' or girls' clubs; and sidewalks or walking paths available in their neighborhood

---

*Some policy and environmental indicators may not be comparable to findings from the *2010 State Indicator Report on Physical Activity* because of changes to the indicator data source

Youth without access to opportunities for physical activity during non-school hours are less likely to be as physically active as their peers.[10-12] Youth in neighborhoods with access to playgrounds, parks, and recreational facilities are more active and were less likely to be overweight or obese than youth with less access to neighborhood infrastructure that supports physical activity.[13] Evidence also suggests that access to parks, playgrounds, and recreation centers may lead to other active behaviors such as biking or walking to a park location.[14]

Percentage of population in a state that live within ½ mile of a park

For both adults and youth, access to places for physical activity can be created or enhanced by having safe, attractive parks in local neighborhoods. People who live closer to parks are more likely to visit parks and be physically active more often than people who live farther away from parks.[15]

2. Enhance Physical Education and Physical Activity in Schools and Child Care Settings

Schools and child care settings can help children be active by requiring quality physical education, recess, and other structured opportunities for age-appropriate physical activity.[16] Guidance can help schools implement initiatives that create supportive environments to increase physical activity in children and adolescents.

State provides guidance on policies for school districts or schools on time spent in moderate- to vigorous-intensity physical activity during physical education class

School-age children and adolescents should participate in at least 60 minutes of physical activity every day.[1] A substantial percentage of students' physical activity can be provided through a comprehensive, multi-component school-based physical activity program.[17] CDC recommends that comprehensive school health programs provide a substantial percentage of each student's recommended daily amount of physical activity in physical education class.[16]

State provides guidance on policies for school districts or schools on recess

The National Association for Sport and Physical Education recommends elementary schools provide all students with at least one daily period of recess for 20 minutes.[18] Daily recess provides students with the opportunity to engage in physical activity. Studies show that recess can contribute to children meeting physical activity guidelines.[19]

State provides guidance on policies for school districts or schools on walking or biking to or from school

When schools are well-located, with safe sidewalks and pedestrian-friendly street crossings, youth are more likely to walk to school.[20-22] The support or promotion of active transport to school can be achieved by a multitude of programs including but not limited to KidsWalk, Walk-to-School, Walking School Bus, and Safe Routes to School. These programs have the potential to increase physical activity among a large number of youth.[5]

State child care regulations align with national standards for moderate- to vigorous-intensity physical activity for preschoolers

In 2007, nearly 55% of children aged 3 to 6 years and not yet in kindergarten were enrolled in center-based child care.[23] Thus, the child care center can be a useful setting to increase physical activity opportunities for children.[17] The *3rd Caring for Our Children: National Health and Safety Performance Standards for Early Care and Education Programs* recommends preschoolers be allowed 90 to 120 minutes of moderate- to vigorous-intensity physical activity per eight-hour day.[24]

3. Street-Scale and Community-Scale Design Policy

The Community Preventive Services Task Force recommends urban design and land use policies and practices that support physical activity in small geographic areas based on sufficient evidence of their effectiveness in increasing physical activity.[25] Street-scale and community-scale urban design and land use policies involve the efforts of urban planners, architects, engineers, developers, and public health professionals to change the physical environment of small geographic areas (i.e., few blocks for street-scale design and several square miles for community-scale design) in ways that support physical activity.[6,25] State- and local-level policies that support physical activity through community and urban design, land use, or creating alternative travel options (e.g., walking, biking, or other non-motorized options) are recommended environmental strategies to increase physical activity.[25] These policies can improve and provide the necessary infrastructure to support physical activity in communities.

State has adopted some form of Complete Streets policy

State-level Complete Streets policies formalize a state's intent to plan, design, and maintain streets so they are safe for all users (e.g., pedestrians, bicyclists, motorists, transit riders, those in wheelchairs) of all ages and abilities.[26] Complete Streets policies can also create options for travel by providing opportunities for active transportation, such as biking and walking. An ideal Complete Streets policy is multi-faceted. It should include a vision statement, specifies all users, applies to new and retrofit projects, makes exceptions specific, is adoptable by all agencies, encourages street connectivity, directs the use of the latest design criteria, complements the context of the community, establishes performance standards, and includes specific implementation steps.[26]

For more information or to provide feedback on the *State Indicator Report on Physical Activity, 2014,* contact DNPAOCommTeam@CDC.gov. Supporting materials for the *State Indicator Report on Physical Activity, 2014,* are available at http://www.cdc.gov/physicalactivity/resources/reports.html

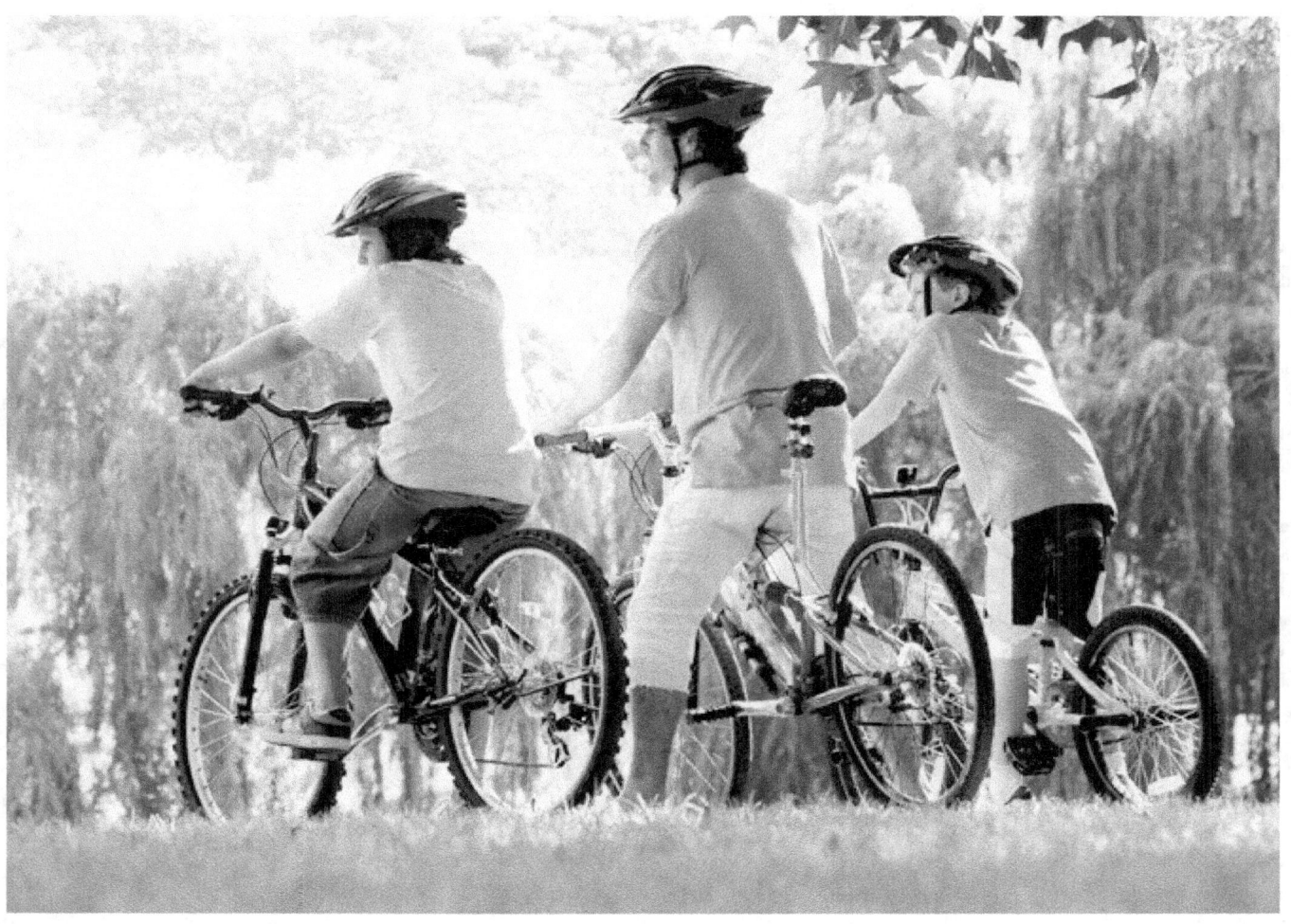

Table 1. State Indicator Report on Physical Activity, 2014, Behavioral Indicators

State	Adults — Percentage(%) who reported						Youth — Percentage (%) who reported		
	No leisure-time physical activity[1]	Met 150 minute aerobic activity guideline[1]	Met 300 minute aerobic activity guideline[1]	Met muscle-strengthening guideline[1]	Met both 150 minute aerobic and muscle-strengthening guidelines	Usually biked or walked to work	No physical activity[2]	Met aerobic activity guideline[2]	Daily physical education[2]
U.S. National	25.4	51.6	31.8	29.3	20.6	3.4	15.2	27.1	29.4
Alabama	32.6	42.4	23.9	24.7	15.0	1.4	20.2	24.8	35.7
Alaska	22.0	57.9	37.7	33.8	25.0	8.9	15.3	20.9	16.0
Arizona	24.1	52.8	33.1	32.5	24.2	3.2	17.3	21.7	23.0
Arkansas	30.9	45.7	27.8	24.7	16.7	2.0	19.9	27.5	23.0
California	19.1	58.2	36.1	32.1	23.7	3.8	N/A	N/A	N/A
Colorado	16.5	61.8	40.7	35.6	27.3	4.3	N/A	N/A	N/A
Connecticut	25.5	52.6	32.8	30.6	21.8	3.3	14.1	26.0	N/A
Delaware	27.0	48.5	28.3	32.3	21.5	2.6	19.1	23.7	13.1
District of Columbia	19.8	57.6	34.4	36.1	26.3	14.8	27.7	16.4	N/A
Florida	26.9	52.8	33.7	29.2	21.4	2.2	18.7	25.3	24.2
Georgia	26.7	50.7	31.8	30.2	20.7	1.8	18.7	24.7	33.6
Hawaii	21.3	58.5	38.1	32.1	23.7	5.8	17.4	22.0	7.3
Idaho	21.4	57.2	35.9	30.3	22.4	4.3	10.8	27.9	22.4
Illinois	25.1	51.7	31.2	31.4	22.0	3.7	12.9	25.4	63.6
Indiana	29.2	46.0	27.5	26.0	17.3	2.6	N/A	N/A	N/A
Iowa	25.9	47.6	26.9	27.5	17.2	4.1	N/A	N/A	N/A
Kansas	26.8	46.8	26.4	24.5	16.5	2.9	14.4	28.3	27.9
Kentucky	29.3	46.8	29.3	26.3	17.3	2.3	19.9	22.5	19.3
Louisiana	33.8	42.0	25.9	23.9	15.5	2.4	N/A	N/A	33.6
Maine	23.0	56.7	35.6	27.5	20.6	4.3	14.0	22.3	4.5
Maryland	26.2	48.7	28.8	30.2	19.8	2.6	18.0	21.6	18.2
Massachusetts	23.5	56.3	35.7	32.0	23.3	5.4	13.2	23.0	16.7
Michigan	23.6	53.5	33.6	28.8	19.7	2.7	15.2	26.7	26.8
Minnesota	21.9	54.0	33.7	29.6	20.9	3.5	N/A	N/A	N/A
Mississippi	36.0	40.0	23.7	23.9	14.2	1.8	22.8	25.9	28.7
Missouri	28.4	49.5	30.5	24.7	17.3	2.2	17.1	27.2	30.9
Montana	24.4	55.3	36.0	30.2	21.8	6.2	10.7	27.7	34.9
Nebraska	26.3	49.0	28.6	28.1	19.0	3.4	10.7	32.3	34.9
Nevada	24.3	52.6	33.8	30.1	21.3	2.4	15.3	24.0	25.9
New Hampshire	22.5	56.1	34.3	30.4	22.3	3.1	11.6	22.9	18.2
New Jersey	26.4	53.2	33.1	31.7	23.1	3.5	11.6	27.6	45.2
New Mexico	25.3	52.2	33.1	31.5	22.3	3.1	12.7	31.1	25.1
New York	26.3	51.5	32.0	30.1	21.5	6.9	15.2	25.7	18.9
North Carolina	26.7	46.8	28.2	27.7	18.3	2.0	17.7	25.9	N/A
North Dakota	27.1	47.3	26.1	27.4	18.0	4.4	10.9	24.7	N/A
Ohio	27.0	51.6	32.9	30.4	21.4	2.6	13.2	25.9	N/A
Oklahoma	31.2	44.8	27.1	23.8	16.2	2.1	13.6	38.5	32.2
Oregon	19.8	61.1	40.7	30.9	23.4	6.2	N/A	N/A	N/A
Pennsylvania	26.2	49.4	29.9	27.8	18.8	4.3	N/A	N/A	N/A
Rhode Island	26.2	48.7	29.1	28.5	19.5	4.0	12.8	23.2	25.7
South Carolina	27.2	50.0	30.6	27.6	18.5	2.3	19.6	23.8	N/A
South Dakota	27.0	46.1	25.3	26.1	16.0	4.8	15.0	27.7	18.5
Tennessee	35.1	39.0	22.7	20.6	12.7	1.5	19.6	25.4	22.3
Texas	27.2	48.2	27.6	28.3	19.0	1.9	16.6	30.0	38.3
Utah	18.9	55.8	33.6	32.3	22.5	3.5	10.0	19.7	18.6
Vermont	21.0	59.2	39.9	29.0	21.6	6.5	13.7	25.4	14.5
Virginia	25.0	52.4	33.6	33.4	22.7	2.7	15.2	23.8	13.3
Washington	22.0	54.2	34.0	30.6	21.0	4.3	N/A	N/A	N/A
West Virginia	35.1	43.0	26.1	20.2	12.7	3.0	15.0	31.0	30.7
Wisconsin	22.7	57.4	35.4	29.2	22.3	4.0	12.6	24.0	39.4
Wyoming	25.5	53.1	33.0	29.6	21.2	4.3	13.9	28.2	23.7

[1] Weighted percentage; [2] National percentage from national YRBSS survey; state percentages from state YRBSS surveys; both are weighted percentages; N/A = Not available.

Table 2. State Indicator Report on Physical Activity, 2014, Policy and Environmental Indicators

	Policy and Environmental Indicators by Strategy							
Strategy	Create or enhance access to safe places for physical activity			Enhance Physical Education and Physical Activity in Schools and Childcare Settings				Support street- and community-scale design policy
				State provided policy guidance on:			State child care regulations meet CFOC Guidelines of moderate- to vigorous-intensity physical activity for preschoolers in all settings	
State	State provided policy guidance on joint-use agreements	% of youth with parks, community centers, and sidewalks in neighborhood*	% of population that live within ½ mile of a park	Time spent in moderate- to vigorous-intensity physical activity in PE	Recess	Walking or biking to/ from school		State adopted some form of Complete Streets policy
U.S. National	20[1]	54.5[2]	39.2	28[1]	30[1]	34[1]	0[1]	27[1]
Alabama	No	37.0	14.7	Yes	No	No	No	No
Alaska	Yes	57.1	41.7	Yes	Yes	Yes	No	No
Arizona	Yes	57.3	38.0	Yes	Yes	Yes	No	No
Arkansas	Yes	43.0	15.3	No	No	No	No	No
California	No	66.7	58.3	Yes	No	Yes	No	Yes
Colorado	Yes	69.9	59.5	Yes	Yes	Yes	No	Yes
Connecticut	Yes	54.7	34.6	Yes	Yes	No	No	Yes
Delaware	No	51.8	46.3	Yes	Yes	Yes	No	Yes
District of Columbia	Yes	76.3	88.1	Yes	Yes	Yes	No	N/A
Florida	No	51.4	30.7	Yes	No	Yes	No	Yes
Georgia	No	41.1	15.1	No	No	No	No	Yes
Hawaii	No	68.0	67.2	Yes	Yes	No	No	Yes
Idaho	No	55.5	36.2	Yes	No	No	No	No
Illinois	No	65.6	58.7	No	Yes	No	No	Yes
Indiana	N/A	47.9	27.1	N/A	No	No	No	No
Iowa	No	58.2	44.5	No	No	No	No	No
Kansas	Yes	59.1	43.0	Yes	Yes	Yes	No	No
Kentucky	Yes	40.6	19.8	Yes	Yes	Yes	No	No
Louisiana	Yes	35.4	22.3	No	No	No	No	Yes
Maine	No	48.7	11.2	Yes	Yes	Yes	No	No
Maryland	No	56.9	50.8	No	No	No	No	Yes
Massachusetts	No	63.2	49.3	No	No	Yes	No	Yes
Michigan	No	52.5	36.9	No	Yes	No	No	Yes
Minnesota	No	60.7	60.3	Yes	Yes	Yes	No	Yes
Mississippi	Yes	30.0	10.9	Yes	No	Yes	No	Yes
Missouri	Yes	50.0	32.8	No	Yes	Yes	No	No
Montana	No	53.7	36.3	No	Yes	Yes	No	No
Nebraska	Yes	56.8	50.1	Yes	Yes	Yes	No	No
Nevada	No	64.6	38.6	Yes	Yes	Yes	No	No
New Hampshire	No	51.2	17.1	No	No	No	No	No
New Jersey	No	59.6	45.1	No	No	Yes	No	Yes
New Mexico	Yes	52.8	37.3	No	No	Yes	No	No
New York	No	57.4	51.6	No	No	No	No	Yes
North Carolina	Yes	41.4	13.5	Yes	Yes	Yes	No	Yes
North Dakota	No	59.8	42.1	Yes	Yes	Yes	No	No
Ohio	No	52.2	40.4	No	No	No	No	No
Oklahoma	No	40.6	33.4	Yes	Yes	Yes	No	No
Oregon	Yes	62.4	54.1	Yes	Yes	Yes	No	Yes
Pennsylvania	No	53.3	35.0	No	No	Yes	No	Yes
Rhode Island	No	64.6	41.0	No	Yes	Yes	No	Yes
South Carolina	No	36.1	12.9	Yes	No	Yes	No	Yes
South Dakota	Yes	58.3	39.3	Yes	Yes	Yes	No	No
Tennessee	Yes	37.0	17.5	No	Yes	Yes	No	Yes
Texas	No	53.1	32.5	Yes	Yes	Yes	No	Yes
Utah	No	69.1	52.5	No	Yes	Yes	No	No
Vermont	No	46.2	13.9	Yes	Yes	Yes	No	Yes
Virginia	Yes	53.1	31.0	Yes	Yes	Yes	No	Yes
Washington	No	61.1	49.3	No	Yes	Yes	No	Yes
West Virginia	Yes	57.2	9.0	Yes	Yes	Yes	No	No
Wisconsin	Yes	33.8	49.4	No	No	No	No	Yes
Wyoming	No	61.8	27.4	No	No	No	No	No

[1] Total Count [2] Mean; N/A = not available * Percentage of youth in a state with parks or playground areas; recreation centers, community centers, or boys' or girls' clubs; and sidewalks or walking paths available in their neighborhood

Indicator Definitions and Data Sources

Adult Behavioral Indicators

- Percentage of adults in the state who engaged in no leisure-time physical activity
- Percentage of adults in the state who met the 150 minute aerobic activity guideline
- Percentage of adults in the state who met the 300 minute aerobic activity guideline
- Percentage of adults in the state who met the muscle-strengthening guideline
- Percentage of adults in the state who met the 150 minute aerobic activity guideline and the muscle-strengthening guideline

Data were derived from Behavioral Risk Factor Surveillance System (BRFSS) (adults aged ≥ 18 years), 2011. Respondents whose physical activity level could not be categorized due to missing physical activity data were excluded. Data are weighted.

> The BRFSS questionnaire is an annual, state-based telephone survey that includes seven (7) questions about non-occupational aerobic physical activity and one question about muscle-strengthening activity on the odd calendar years. The questions are preceded by the following statement: "The next few questions are about exercise, recreation, or physical activities other than your regular job duties." Respondents who report "no" to participating in any physical activities or exercises such as running, calisthenics, golf, gardening, or walking for exercise during the past month were classified as engaging in no leisure-time activity. Respondents who report "yes" to participating in any leisure-time physical activities during the past month are then asked about their participation in other aerobic physical activities. To determine the percentage of adults that meet aerobic physical activity guidelines, respondents are asked to report the frequency and duration of the two aerobic physical activities at which they spent the most time during the past month or week. Respondents are classified as meeting the aerobic physical activity guideline if they report at least 150 minutes per week of moderate-intensity aerobic activity, or at least 75 minutes of vigorous-intensity aerobic activity, or an equivalent combination of moderate- and vigorous-intensity aerobic activity (where vigorous-intensity minutes are multiplied by 2) totaling at least 150 minutes per week. Respondents are classified as meeting the 300 minute

aerobic guideline if they report more than 300 minutes per week of moderate-intensity aerobic activity, or more than 150 minutes per week of vigorous-intensity aerobic activity, or an equivalent combination of moderate- and vigorous-intensity aerobic activity (where vigorous-intensity minutes are multiplied by 2) totaling greater than 300 minutes per week.[1]

To determine the percentage of adults that participate in muscle-strengthening activities, respondents are asked to report the frequency of their participation in activities to strengthen their muscles during the past month or week. Respondents are classified as meeting the muscle-strengthening guideline, if they report participating in muscle-strengthening activities at least 2 times per week. Respondents are classified as meeting both the aerobic and muscle-strengthening guidelines if they met 1) the aerobic physical activity guideline and 2) the muscle-strengthening guideline.

Survey questions and data are available at: http://www.cdc.gov/ brfss/questionnaires/pdf-ques/2011brfss.pdf and http://www. cdc.gov/brfss/annual_data/annual_2011.htm Accessed August 12, 2013. Additional guidance on how to assess the *2008 Physical Activity Guidelines for Americans* using 2011 BRFSS data is available at: http:// wwwdev.cdc.gov/brfss/pdf/PA%20RotatingCore_BRFSSGuide_50 8Comp_07252013FINAL.pdf Accessed September 13, 2013.

Percentage of adults in the state who usually biked or walked to work in the last week

Data derived from the U.S. Census Bureau, American Community Survey 2009–2011, (persons aged ≥ 16 years).

The U.S. Census Bureau's American Community Survey is an ongoing, annual survey of a percentage of the U.S. population. This report used the journey to work question that asks, "How did this person usually get to work last week?" Respondents who reported, "Bicycle'" or "Walked" were classified as usually biked or walked to work.

Data and survey questions are available at http://www.census. gov/acs/www/about_the_survey/american_community_survey/ Accessed August 12, 2013.

Youth Behavioral Indicators

- Percentage of students in grades 9–12 in the state who did not engage in at least 60 minutes of physical activity on any day

- Percentage of students in grades 9–12 in the state who met the aerobic activity guideline

- Percentage of students in grades 9–12 in the state who engaged in daily school physical education

Data derived from the Youth Risk Behavior Surveillance System (YRBSS), 2013 (students in grades 9–12). Respondents with missing data were excluded. Data are weighted.

The 2013 YRBSS questionnaire included three (3) questions about physical activity and two (2) questions about physical education asked via a classroom survey. This report uses the questions specific to time spent in moderate- to vigorous-intensity physical activity and daily physical education. Respondents were classified as not engaging in any physical activity if they answered "0 days" to the following question: "During the past 7 days, on how many days were you physically active for a total of at least 60 minutes per day? (Add up all the time you spent in any kind of physical activity that increased your heart rate and made you breathe hard some of the time.)" Respondents were classified as meeting the youth aerobic guideline if they answered, "7 days", to the same question. Respondents were classified as engaging in daily school physical education if they answered "5 days" to the following question: "In an average week when you are in school, on how many days do you go to physical education (PE) classes?"

The national estimate was derived from the national Youth Risk Behavior Survey, conducted among a nationally representative sample of students in grades 9–12. The state estimates were derived from Youth Risk Behavior Surveys conducted among representative samples of students in grades 9–12 in each state. Some states may not have estimates for participation in physical activity or physical education among adolescents. This may be due to either not collecting survey data, not achieving a high enough overall response rate to receive weighted results, or omitting one or more questionnaire items during administration of the survey. Muscle-strengthening data was not collected at the state level and therefore, not eligible for inclusion in this report.

Survey questions and data are available at: http://www.cdc.gov/healthyyouth/yrbs/pdf/questionnaire/2013_hs_questionnaire.pdf and http://www.cdc.gov/healthyyouth/yrbs/data/index.htm Accessed June 17, 2014.

Policy and Environmental Indicators

The definitions for the eight policy and environmental indicators are described below.

State provides guidance on policies for school districts or schools on joint-use agreements for physical activity facilities

Data were derived from CDC's 2012 School Health Policies and Practices Study (SHPPS). SHPPS is a national survey conducted every six (6) years to assess school health policies and practices at the state, district, school, and classroom levels. This indicator used one (1) question from the SHPPS Physical Education and Physical Activity state questionnaire.

States where the state education agency personnel answered, "Yes", to the question, "During the past two years, did your state distribute or provide model policies, policy guidance, or other materials to inform district or school policy on joint-use agreements for physical activity facilities?," were classified as providing guidance on policies for school districts or schools on joint-use agreements for physical activity facilities.

Survey questions and data are available at: http://www.cdc.gov/healthyyouth/shpps/index.htm Accessed September 4, 2013.

Percentage of youth in a state with parks or playground areas; recreation centers, community centers, or boys' or girls' clubs; and sidewalks or walking paths available in their neighborhood

Data were derived from the 2011–2012 National Survey of Children's Health (NSCH), (Youth age > 17 years old). This indicator used questions from the Neighborhood and Community Characteristics section of the survey.

Parents of youth who answered "Yes" to all of the following questions, "Please tell me if the following places and things are available to children in your neighborhood, even if [CHILD'S NAME] does not actually use them: 1) park or playground area? 2) a recreation center, community center, or boys' or girls' club? 3) sidewalks or walking paths? ," were classified as having parks or playground areas; recreation centers, community centers, or boys' or girls' clubs; and sidewalks or walking paths available in their neighborhood.

Survey questions and methods are available at: http://childhealthdata.org/learn/methods. Survey data are available by request at: http://childhealthdata.org/help/dataset. Accessed August 16, 2013.

Percentage of population in a state that live within ½ mile of a park

Data were derived from the CDC's National Environmental Public Health Tracking Network (Tracking Network), a system of integrated health, exposure, and hazard information and data from a variety of national, state, and city sources. This indicator uses the park access data reported in the Community Design section of the Tracking Network.

To determine the population in a state living within ½ mile of a park, the Tracking Network used two (2) data sources, NAVTEQ and the U.S. Census Bureau. NAVTEQ 2010 mapping data on national, state, and local parks were used to locate park boundaries. The 2010 U.S. Census Bureau census and Topologically Integrated Geographic Encoding and Referencing (TIGER) mapping data were used to obtain census state- and block-level population and boundaries. Using geospatial analysis software, a ½-mile buffer was created around each park. The percentage of the area of each block that fell within park buffers was multiplied by the block's population to estimate the block-level population residing within ½ mile of a park. The population that lives within ½ mile of a park was summed over all blocks in a state to estimate the total population of the state that lives within ½ mile of a park.

Census data can be found at http://www2.census.gov/census_2010/04-Summary_File_1/. Tracking Network data are available at: http://ephtracking.cdc.gov/showCommunityDesign.action. Accessed August 8, 2013.

State provides guidance on policies for school districts or schools on time spent in moderate- to vigorous-intensity physical activity during physical education class

Data were derived from the 2012 SHPPS. This indicator used one question from the SHPPS Physical Education and Physical Activity state questionnaire.

States where the state education agency personnel answered "Yes" to the question, "During the past two years, did your state distribute or provide model policies, policy guidance, or other materials to inform district or school policy on time spent in moderate- to vigorous-intensity physical activity during physical education class?," were classified as providing guidance on policies for school districts or schools on time spent in moderate- to vigorous-intensity physical activity during physical education class.

Survey questions and data are available at: http://www.cdc.gov/healthyyouth/shpps/index.htm. Accessed September 4, 2013.

State provides guidance on policies for school districts or schools on recess

Data were derived from the 2012 SHPPS. This indicator used one question from the SHPPS Physical Education and Physical Activity state questionnaire.

States where the state education agency personnel answered "Yes" to the question, "During the past two years, did your state distribute or provide model policies, policy guidance, or other materials to inform district or school policy on recess?," were classified as providing guidance on policies for school districts or schools on recess.

Survey questions and data are available at http://www.cdc.gov/healthyyouth/shpps/index.htm. Accessed September 4, 2013.

State provides guidance on policies for school districts or schools on walking or biking to or from school

Data were derived from the 2012 SHPPS. This indicator used one question from the SHPPS Physical Education and Physical Activity state questionnaire.

States where the state education agency personnel answered "Yes" to the question, "During the past two years, did your state distribute or provide model policies, policy guidance, or other materials to inform district or school policy on walking or biking to or from school?," were classified as providing guidance on policies for school districts or schools on walking or biking to or from school.

Survey questions and data are available at http://www.cdc.gov/healthyyouth/shpps/index.htm. Accessed September 4, 2013.

State child care regulations align with national standards for moderate- to vigorous-intensity physical activity for preschoolers

Data were derived from the 2012 National Resource Center for Health and Safety in Child Care and Early Education (NRC). This indicator used NRC's analysis of the degree to which state child care regulations for licensed child care center types (1) child care centers, (2) large or group family child care homes, and (3) small family child care homes reflect national standards for moderate-to vigorous-intensity physical activity for preschoolers as described in the 3rd *Caring for Our Children: National Health and Safety Performance Standards for Early Care and Education Programs.* The standards (section 3.1.3.1) specify that preschoolers should be allowed 90 to 120 minutes of moderate- to vigorous-intensity physical activity per eight-hour day.

States with regulations fully addressing standards for all three licensed child care types were designated as "yes." States with regulations that did not fully address standards in any child care type were designated as "no."

National Resource Center for Health and Safety in Child Care and Early Education. Achieving a State of Healthy Weight: 2012 Update. Aurora, CO: NRC. Data are available at: http://nrckids.org/default/assets/File/ASHW%202012%20Final%20Report%207-24-13.pdf. Accessed August 12, 2013.

State has adopted some form of Complete Streets policy

Data were derived from the National Complete Streets Coalition's 2012 policy analysis. The National Complete Streets Coalition issues regular reports and guidance on Complete Streets policy to provide examples and support to states and communities looking to adopt new policies.

States that adopted a state-level Complete Streets policy before December 13, 2012, were given a "yes." The state policy number, key policy language, and a link to the state policy are available at http://www.smartgrowthamerica.org/documents/cs/policy/cs-state-policies.pdf. Accessed August 12, 2013.

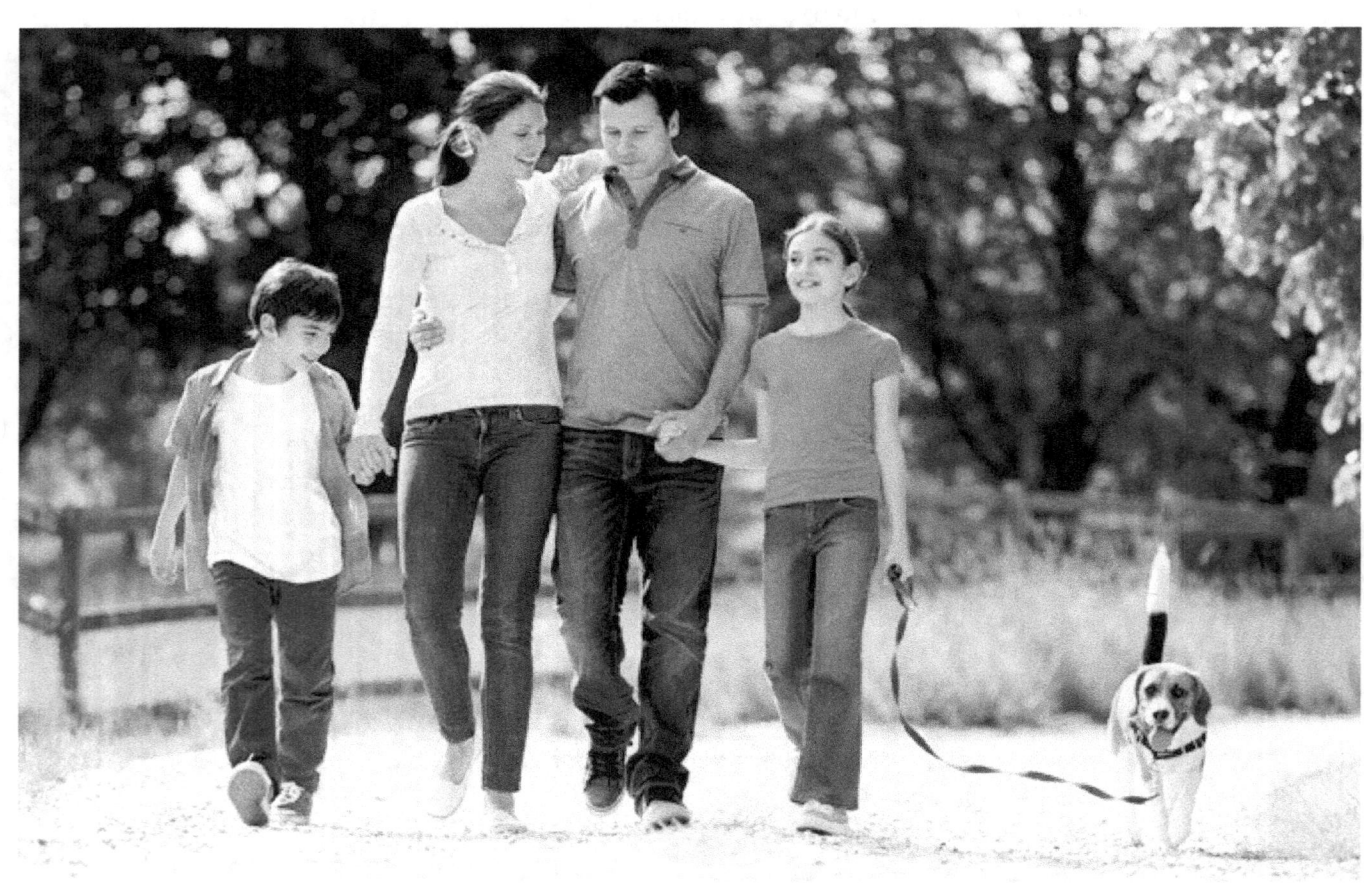

References

1. U S. Department of Health and Human Services. 2008 Physical Activity Guidelines for Americans. In: U S. Department of Health and Human Services, editor. Hyattsville, MD2008.

2. Physical Activity Guidelines Advisory Committee. Physical Activity Guidelines Advisory Committee Report, 2008. In: U.S. Department of Health and Human Services, editor. Washington, DC2008.

3. Centers for Disease Control and Prevention. Adult Participation in Aerobic and Muscle-Strengthening Physical Activities—United States, 2011. Morb Mortal Wkly Rep. 2013;62(No.RR-17):326-30.

4. Centers for Disease Control and Prevention. Youth Risk Behavior Surveillance, United States, 2011. Morb Mortal Wkly Rep. 2012;61(No. SS-4):1-28.

5. Centers for Disease Control and Prevention. Strategies to Prevent Obesity and Other Chronic Diseases: The CDC Guide to Strategies for Increasing Physical Activity in the Community. In: U.S. Department of Health and Human Services, editor. Atlanta 2011.

6. Kahn E, Ramsey L, Brownson R, al. e. The effectiveness of interventions to increase physical activity: A systematic review. Am J Prev Med. 2002;22(4 suppl):73-107.

7. Pate R. A national physical activity plan for the United States. J Phys Act Health. 2009;Nov(6 suppl 2):S157-S8.

8. U S. Department of Health and Human Services Office of Disease Prevention and Health Promotion. Healthy People 2020. Washington, DC.

9. Evenson K, Wen F, Lee S, Heinrich K, Eyer A. National study of changes in community access to school physical activity facilities: The School Health Polices and Programs Study. J Phys Act Health. 2010;7(suppl 1):S20-S30.

10. Cohen D, Ashwood J, Scott M, Overton A, Evenson K, Staten L, et al. Public parks and physical activity among adolescent girls. Pediatrics. 2006;188:e1381-e9.

11. Roemmich J, Epstein L, Raja S, Yin L, Robinson J, Winiewicz D. Association of access to parks and recreational facilities with the physical activity of young children. Prev Med. 2006;43(6):437-41.

12. Epstein L, Raja S, Gold S, Paluch R, Pak Y, Roemmich J. Reducing sedentary behavior: the relationship between park area and physical activity of youth. Psychol Sci. 2006;17(8):654-9.

13. Veugelers P, Sithole F, Zhang S, Muhajarine N. Neighborhood characteristics in relation to diet, physical activity and overweight of Canadian children. Int J Pediatr Obes. 2008;3:152-9.

14. Grow H, Saelens B, Kerr J, Durant N, Norman G, Sallis J. Where are youth active? Roles of proximity, active transport and build environment. Med Sci Sports Exerc. 2008;40(12):2071-9.

15. Cohen DA, McKenzie TL, al. e. Contribution of public parks to physical activity American Journal of Public Health. 2007;97(3):509-14.

16. Center for Disease Control and Prevention. School Health Guide to Promote Healthy Eating and Physical Activity. Morb Mortal Wkly Rep. 2011;60(No.RR-5):1-80.

17. Physical Activity Guidelines for Americans Midcourse Report Subcommittee of the President's Council on Fitness SN. Physical Activity Guidelines for Americans Midcourse Report: Strategies to Increase Physical Activity Among Youth,. In: U.S. Department of Health and Human Services, editor. Washington, D.C.2012.

18. National Association for Sport and Physical Education. Recess in Elementary Schools. Reston,VA: National Association for Sport and Physical Education, 2006.

19. Ridgers N, Stratton G, Fairclough S. Physical activity levels of children during school playtime. Sports Med. 2006;36(4):359-71.

20. Tudor-Locke C, Ainsworth B, Popkin B. Active commuting to school: An overlooked source of children's physical activity? Sports Med. 2001;31(5):309-13.

21. Zhu X, Lee C. Correlates of Walking to School and Implications of Public Policies: Survey Results from Parents of Elementary School Children in Austin, Texas Journal of Public Health Policy, . 2009;30:S177-S202.

22. National Safe Routes to School Taskforce. Safe routes to school: a transportation legacy. A national strategy to increase safety and physical activity among American youth. Chapel Hill, NC 2008.

23. Federal Interagency Forum on Child and Family Statistics. America's Children: Key National Indicators of Well-Being, 2013. Washington, DC: U S. Government Printing Office; 2013

24. American Academy of Pediatrics, American Public Health Association, National Resource Center for Health and Safety in Child Care and Early Education. Caring for our children: National health and safety performance standards; Guidelines for early care and education programs. Elk Grove Village, IL Washington, DC.: American Academy of Pediatrics American Public Health Association., 2011.

25. Heath G, Brownson R, Kruger J, Miles R, Powell K, Ramsey L. The effectiveness of urban design and land use and transport policies and practices to increase physical activity: A systematic review. J Phys Act Health. 2006;3(suppl 1):S55-S76.

26. Seskin S, McCann B. Complete Streets Local Policy Workbook. Smart Growth America, National Complete Streets Coalition., 2012.